WHAT DID JESUS EAT?

By Anne Skinner

Hannah House Publishing
MPO Box 2813,
Niagara Falls, New York, 14302

ISBN-13: 978-1511589406
ISBN-10: 151158940X

INTRODUCTION

Approximately four years ago I started to think of the many foods that Jesus would have eaten.
Living in Canada and USA most of my life I just assumed that He would eat what we ate, which is so wrong. I decided that the only way to find out this was to start doing some research on His life, His family and the foods that He would have eaten and also what He would want us to eat.

The more I did research the more I got intrigued with the types of food and their benefits for our body.

I realized more and more that the Bible actually gave us a good description on how to eat healthy and stay healthy.

I have put this book together to help you to understand better the diet of Jesus and how we should follow in His Footsteps not just in our daily life of living but in what we eat too.

BASIC BIBLE EATING

From the book of Genesis to Revelations, the Bible makes several references to food. Genesis 1:29 reads, "I have given you every plant yielding seed, which is upon the face of the Earth and every tree with seed in its fruit; you shall have them for food" - God's instruction to Adam. In Deuteronomy 8:8, the Israelites are promised "a good land ... , a land of wheat and barley, of vines, figs, and pomegranates, a land of olive trees and honey".

Beliefnet.com provides insights on seven healthy foods from the Bible. This provides the basis for eating healthy. According to Beliefnet.com, the ancients might not have known the word 'antioxidant', but they were into eating 'super-foods'.

Apples

Song of Solomon 2:5 - Strengthen me with raisins, refresh me with apples, for I am faint with love. Apples contain insoluble fibre which is helpful for constipation and protection against colon cancer. Rich in pectin, a fibre that controls cholesterol, apples are rich in vitamin C for the immune system and healing wounds. Apples are also rich in boron, a mineral that boosts alertness.

Wheat

Ezekiel 4:9 - Take wheat and barley, beans and lentils, millet and spelt; put them in a storage jar and use them to make bread for yourself. You are to eat it during the 390 days you lie on your side - (healingscripture.com). As a grain, wheat is used in the production of almost anything - from bread to

pasta to cakes. It is healthiest when unrefined. Wholewheat products are high in fibre, contributing 30 per cent of the recommended daily intake. Wheat also provides high levels of manganese and magnesium. A wheat- rich diet increases energy levels and reduces the risk of type-2 diabetes, gallstones and other diseases.

Barley

Deuteronomy 8:8 - For the Lord your God is bringing you into a good land with wheat and barley, vines and fig trees, pomegranates, olive oil and honey.
Barley is another wholesome grain that is used in the preparation of breads and cereals and hearty soups. The high fibre content in barley makes it good for maintaining intestinal health, lowering cholesterol and reducing the risk of colon cancer and type-2 diabetes. Symptoms of arthritis can be reduced through the trace amounts of copper in barley.

Grapes

Numbers 13:23 - When they reached the Valley of Eshcol, they cut off a branch bearing a single cluster of grapes. Two of them carried it on a pole between them, along with some pomegranates and figs. Grapes produce grape juice, red wine and raisins, all of which are healthy because grapes are rich in flavonoids, which are believed to reduce your risk of blood clots and protect your body from damage by the 'free radicals' found in LDL, or 'bad', cholesterol. Antioxidants are abundant in grapes, providing protection against cardiovascular disease, particularly in women.

Figs

1 Samuel 30:11-12 - They found an Egyptian in a field and brought him to David ... . They gave him water to drink and food to eat ... part of a cake of pressed figs and two cakes of raisins. He ate and was revived, for he had not eaten any food or drunk any water for three days and three nights.

Figs are eaten either dried or fresh and are high in potassium, which is important to blood-pressure control. A rich source of dietary fibre, figs also contain calcium, which can help preserve bone density, and B vitamins for a healthy skin. The extract from fig leaves helps to lower insulin levels in diabetics. Interestingly, early olympians wore figs as a sign of honour. Figs are now part of the Olympic symbols.

Pomegranates

Deuteronomy 8:8 - a land with wheat and barley, vines and fig trees, pomegranates, olive oil and honey.

These sweet fruits, eaten either dried or fresh, are rich in potassium, a mineral that helps control blood pressure, reducing the risk of stroke and circulatory disease. They are also high in dietary fibre, which may help you lose weight, and they are a fruit source of calcium, which can help preserve bone density. Fig leaves, which are not typically eaten but can be made into an extract, are thought to help lower insulin levels in diabetics.

Pomegranates are suitable for edible garnishes, soups, salad, meats and desserts.

Olive oil

Numbers 18:12 - all the best of the fresh oil and all the best of the fresh wine and of the grain, the first fruits of those which they give to the Lord, I give them to you.

Olive oil, made from pressing olives, particularly the extra-virgin product which is the finest product, contains an abundance of the antioxidants that control high cholesterol. Of importance too, are the high amounts of monounsaturated fatty acids which have been shown to reduce total cholesterol but raising 'good' cholesterol levels, keeping the arteries free from plaque. High in vitamin E, olive oil can protect against colon cancer and will reduce the conditions associated with gastritis and other stomach ailments.

Seasonings, Spices and Herbs

•Anise (Matthew 23:23 KJV)
•Coriander (Exodus 16:31; Numbers 11:7)
•Cinnamon (Exodus 30:23; Revelation 18:13)
•Cumin (Isaiah 28:25; Matthew 23:23)
•Dill (Matthew 23:23)
•Garlic (Numbers 11:5)
•Mint (Matthew 23:23; Luke 11:42)
•Mustard (Matthew 13:31)
•Rue (Luke 11:42)
•Salt (Ezra 6:9; Job 6:6)

Fruits and Nuts

•Apples (Song of Solomon 2:5)
•Almonds (Genesis 43:11; Numbers 17:8)
•Dates (2 Samuel 6:19; 1 Chronicles 16:3)
•Figs (Nehemiah 13:15; Jeremiah 24:1-3)
•Grapes (Leviticus 19:10; Deuteronomy 23:24)
•Melons (Numbers 11:5; Isaiah 1:8)
•Olives (Isaiah 17:6; Micah 6:15)
•Pistachio Nuts (Genesis 43:11)
•Pomegranates (Numbers 20:5; Deuteronomy 8:8)
•Raisins (Numbers 6:3; 2 Samuel 6:19)
•Sycamore Fruit (Psalm 78:47; Amos 7:14)

Vegetables and Legumes

•Beans (2 Samuel 17:28; Ezekiel 4:9)
•Cucumbers (Numbers 11:5)
•Gourds (2 Kings 4:39)

•Leeks (Numbers 11:5)
•Lentils (Genesis 25:34; 2 Samuel 17:28; Ezekiel 4:9)
•Onions (Numbers 11:5)

Grains

•Barley (Deuteronomy 8:8; Ezekiel 4:9)
•Bread (Genesis 25:34; 2 Samuel 6:19; 16:1; Mark 8:14)
•Corn (Matthew 12:1; KJV - refers to "grain" such as wheat or barley)
•Flour (2 Samuel 17:28; 1 Kings 17:12)
•Millet (Ezekiel 4:9)
•Spelt (Ezekiel 4:9)
•Unleavened Bread (Genesis 19:3; Exodus 12:20)
•Wheat (Ezra 6:9; Deuteronomy 8:8)

Fish

•Matthew 15:36
•John 21:11-13

Fowl

•Partridge (1 Samuel 26:20; Jeremiah 17:11)
•Pigeon (Genesis 15:9; Leviticus 12:8)
•Quail (Psalm 105:40)
•Dove (Leviticus 12:8)

Animal Meats

- Calf (Proverbs 15:17; Luke 15:23)
- Goat (Genesis 27:9)
- Lamb (2 Samuel 12:4)
- Oxen (1 Kings 19:21)
- Sheep (Deuteronomy 14:4)
- Venison (Genesis 27:7 KJV)

Dairy

- Butter (Proverbs 30:33)
- Cheese (2 Samuel 17:29; Job 10:10)
- Curds (Isaiah 7:15)
- Milk (Exodus 33:3; Job 10:10; Judges 5:25)

Miscellaneous

- Eggs (Job 6:6; Luke 11:12)
- Grape Juice (Numbers 6:3)
- Honey (Exodus 33:3; Deuteronomy 8:8; Judges 14:8-9)
- Locust (Mark 1:6)
- Olive Oil (Ezra 6:9; Deuteronomy 8:8)
- Vinegar (Ruth 2:14; John 19:29)
- Wine (Ezra 6:9; John 2:1-10)

BIBLE INFORMATION REGARDING OUR DIET...

7 Food Rainbow Colors Bible Dieting is simple. The foods are color coded.

Rainbow Foods

Our food was created to be appealing to all of our senses - especially our senses
of taste, smell and sight. Within the skin pigments and edible portion of these
living foods lies a vast array of phytonutrients most of which have yet to be fully understood or documented by science. Be joyful and eat for abundant life.

Red Foods

Trees: cherries, apples, cranberries, papaya, pomegranate Plants: tomatoes, strawberries, watermelon, raspberries Herbs: beets, rhubarb, radishes
Nutrient: Lycopene

Orange Foods

Trees: oranges, grapefruit, peaches
Plants: pumpkin, squash
Herbs: carrots, sweet potatoes, yams Nutrient: beta-carotene

Yellow Foods

Trees: lemons, pears, apricots, grapefruit Plants: corn, Squash, wheat, cantaloupe Herbs: rutabagas
Nutrient: vitamin C

Green Foods

Trees: avocados, olives, pears, lime
Plants: cucumbers, peas, green beans, zucchini
Herbs: broccoli, asparagus, greens, spinach, brussels sprouts, kale, celery, green onions.
Nutrient: lutein

Blue Foods

Plants: blueberries, blackberries, mulberries
Nutrient:
Anthoocyanin

White Foods

Trees: coconut, dates, pears, nuts
Plants: white beans, oats
Herbs: onions, cauliflower, garlic, horseradish, potatoes, turnips, mushrooms, parsnips, shallots, ginger
Nutrient: Allicin
Purple Foods:
Trees: plumbs, prunes, figs
Plants: grapes, blackberries, elderberries

Herbs: beets, eggplants, cabbage

Bible Foods and the Pyramid

The Bible diet pyramid displays the relevant merit of the four Bible food groups. Although we should eat more vegetables and herbs by volume, the nobler tree foods nearer the base are more highly esteemed and hold the greater priority when planning meals.

These three plant food groups follow the order of mention in the creation account as well as the subsequent order in which they were given to mankind for food.

The biblical diet plan may seem similar to vegetarian, kosher, halal or vegan diets. However, not all fruit and vegetables are equal. A hierarchy of food relevance is established based on how seeds are propagated within the tree, plant or herb. Each of the three groups of plant food are distinctly individual and satisfy differing nutritional and health needs. We sometimes use the terms fruit and vegetable loosely to describe plant foods, but the Bible makes a clear distinction.

The Bible health plan indicates that fruit, vegetables, nuts, whole grains and legumes are the foundation of a healthy diet. Herbs, exercise, water and sunshine are also essential for happiness. Safe, clean meat; meat by- products and vegetable oils are optional.

Original Diet - Biblical Diet Foods

The Bible Diet Solution

We want to eat right, but who is the authority on eating right? Dietary experts often disagree. Fad diets come and go, and the science of nutrition can be overwhelming. So who can we trust?

The Bible holds the solution. Before Man was formed, The Lord had already provided for his diet. God created our foods to empower us to bring our noblest ambitions to fruition. His foods are an exact match to our needs.

They were made specifically with mankind in mind. If we know God's simple, trustworthy guidelines, the science of diet will fall into place naturally.

Presented here are simple, biblical principles granted by The Creator through scripture. If our diet is bible based, years of careless living and abuse to our bodies can be reversed in great measure. Damage to our cells can be repaired. Even our healthy appearance can be restored day by day.

Many times as a child I would say to my mother. "Mom, what is God's Will for my life?" She would tell me to read the Bible... I never quite understood it back then but as time went on I saw that in the Bible it was a Roadmap that we could use in our everyday life. Eating was just part of it.

In The Beginning

If we review the first couple chapters of Genesis, we see that each day of creation was a provision for what would be created in succeeding days.

On the third day of creation, the variety of vegetation that covers the earth was spoken into existence. The benefits that plants provide to our planet are countless. For example, the roots of vegetation hold together the soil. With the help of sunshine and rain, plants absorb carbon dioxide and supply fresh oxygen for breathing and natural sugars for the birds and bees. The foliage and flora provide us with both calming and exhilarating spectacles of raw beauty. Yet I say to you that not even Solomon in all his glory clothed himself like one of these. Matthew 6:29.

A principal reason that God created plant life was to provide a replenishable source of food for man and beast. Although it became permissible to eat meat after the great flood, it can be truly stated that plants and plant yield are the purest biblical foods.

You May Freely Eat

And God said, Behold, I have given you every herb yielding seed, which is upon the face of all the earth, and every tree, in which is the fruit of a tree yielding seed; to you it shall be for food. Genesis 1:29
And to every beast of the earth, and to every fowl of the air, and to everything that creepeth upon the earth, wherein there is life, I have given every green herb for meat: and it was so. Genesis 1:30
There are two classes contained within this group for mankind:
1.Every tree yielding seed
Examples: apples, avocados, grapefruit, pecans, papaya, cherries, olives, walnuts
2.Every plant yielding seed
Examples: tomatoes, beans, lentils, wheat, berries, squash, corn, rye

Generally, this diet consists of nuts, grains, legumes, fruits and vegetables. These foods are still the most beneficial to us. Everyday, discoveries in science point to these foods as superior to others for human health and well-being. Seldom does one ever hear a negative report on any of these. If we do, perhaps the report is questionable and not the foods from these groups.

Actually, whenever the results of a new study regarding nutrition is released, it is wise to be skeptical and examine the source and funding for the study. Often, there may be tremendous economic or even political pressures for such studies to have a predetermined outcome.

Take, for example, the changes in the USDA recommendations regarding nutrition over the years. Many of us remember the "four basic food groups" chart developed in 1956. The poster depicting these groups was often prominently displayed in school cafeterias, health classes, clinics etc. The four groups were the meat group, the dairy group, the grain group and the fruits and vegetables group. The image suggested that each group merited equal consideration. This chart was a product of concessions to powerful special interest groups of the time. The meat, dairy and sugar industries were largely instrumental in developing these recommendations. It is obvious to us now. We may not eat freely of all these. Obesity, diabetes, cancer and other diseases are common maladies in our society as a result.

The four food groups standard has been replaced by the food pyramid chart. Although many of the pyramid recommendations are a step in the right direction, they fall far short of the biblical diet plan for the same reasons.

Dietary Restrictions

When God created our dietary system, He had clear lesson plans in mind. As the wind rustles through the leaves of the trees, and the morning dew settles on the tender blades of grass, the science of spiritual edification is whispered to the recesses of our minds. In the second chapter of Genesis, we see God's health plan for man. God placed Adam in a natural setting with nutritional foods, crystal clear waters and responsible work to stimulate his mind and exercise his body. However, man does not live by bread alone. Daily, God walked, talked and communed with Adam and his wife. These simple principles are the foundation on which human happiness is based. God gave Adam access to the tree of life which was in the center of the garden of Eden. He also placed the tree of the knowledge of good and evil in the garden for a special purpose.

The LORD God planted a garden toward the east, in Eden; and there He placed the man whom He had formed. Out of the ground the LORD God caused to grow every tree that is pleasing to the sight and good for food; the tree of life also in the midst of the garden, and the tree of the knowledge of good and evil. Now a river flowed out of Eden to water the garden; and from there it divided and became four rivers. Genesis 2:8-10

Then the LORD God took the man and put him into the garden of Eden to cultivate it and keep it. Genesis 2:15

Every intelligent creature has always possessed the power of choice. Serving God and making right choices has never been compulsory. God does not make robots. On the contrary, by exercising this freedom of choice, our foreheads are broadened and our characters developed. For Adam, obedience to God's law was not a sorrowful duty. It was his natural impulse prompted by reason. These were the days "when the morning stars sang together And all the sons of God shouted for joy" Job 38:7. His dietary boundaries were not confining at all. However, a firm restriction was given to Adam concerning his diet. The LORD God commanded the man, saying, "From any tree of the garden you may eat freely; but from the tree of the knowledge of good and evil you shall not eat, for in the day that you eat from it you will surely die". Genesis 2:17

Controlling our diet is one of the great challenges we encounter in life. There are many accounts in scripture where failure to control appetite has brought about ruin. For example, Adam, Esau, Belshazzar and others have failed in this area with tragic results. Today, those who would be disciplined in diet face tremendous obstacles. The food industry has thrived by producing addictive albeit unhealthy products. Grocery store shelves are filled with delicacies that are a delight to the eyes. Through indulgence, many of us have become subject to our inherited and conditioned unnatural cravings. Thankfully, we can turn things around. Not everyone likes every fruit or vegetable, but there are many varieties of fruits and vegetables available.

Although we eat what we like, it goes beforehand that we like what we eat. We develop tastes for the foods that are familiar. Chinese people love

Chinese foods because they have become accustomed to them. People who live near the Mediterranean Sea love the Mediterranean diet. The same can be said of indigenous diets throughout the world. Humans are highly adaptable creatures. Here is our great advantage when considering biblical dietary reform. We can train our pallets to desire the foods we reasonably choose. Wholesome dieting may take some time and effort to accomplish.

Changing old habits always requires an exercise of our will for awhile. We can take comfort. With perseverance, making healthy dietary choices will become desirable and natural to us in a reasonably short time. This is how sanctification works. We are restored by a renewing of the mind.

The Bible and Herbs

Plants of the field

After Adam's fall, he no longer was privileged to the tree of life. Although his diet had been created to satisfy his nutritional needs, apparently, there were restorative and healing properties associated with the tree of life.
Without the fruit and leaves from this tree, Adam and his offspring would eventually die. In vision, on the island of Patmos, the disciple John saw this tree in the new earth to come. Here is his description:
In the middle of its street. On either side of the river was the tree of life, bearing twelve kinds of fruit, yielding its fruit every month; and the leaves of the tree were for the healing of the nations. Revelation 22:2 (see Ezekiel 47:12)

Then to Adam He said, "Because you have listened to the voice of your wife, and have eaten from the tree about which I commanded you, saying, 'You shall not eat from it'; Cursed is the ground because of you; In toil you will eat of it All the days of your life. "Both thorns and thistles it shall grow for you; And you will eat the plants of the field; By the sweat of your face You will eat bread, Till you return to the ground, Because from it you were taken; For you are dust, And to dust you shall return." Genesis 3:17-19 therefore the LORD God sent him out from the garden of Eden, to cultivate the ground from which he was taken. So He drove the man out; and at the east of the garden of Eden He stationed the Cherubims, and a flaming sword which turned every way, to keep the way of the tree of life. Genesis 3:23-24

Man's diet has been modified to include leafy vegetables and herbs whose seed is not contained inside or the actual edible yield. Here is the modified food groups:
1.Every tree yielding seed
Examples: apples, avocados, grapefruit, pecans, papaya
2.Every plant yielding seed
Examples: tomatoes, beans, lentils, wheat, berries, squash
3.Plants of the field
Examples: greens, onions, parsley, cabbage, celery

Now, man would responsible for planting and cultivating his own food. The ground had been cursed on his behalf making his existence more arduous. Also, he would have to contend with thorns and thistles. These changes weren't intended to be a punishment for sin. Make no mistake. "The wages of sin is death." Rom. 6:23. This curse was yoked to another man who immediately stepped into Adam's place. God's motive for this sacrifice is expressed in the words of The Redeemer. I am come that they might have life, and that they might have life more abundantly". John 10:10. Rather, instead of a curse, these changes were made for man's preservation. For the first time, mankind was exposed to disease and death. The herbs of the field and other vegetables were added to his diet as supplements for health purposes.

Throughout history and throughout the world, herbs have been recognized for their nutritional and medicinal value. Every continent has developed an herbology.

In biblical times, herbs were considered so valuable that they were often used as currency. Everyone should become familiar with basic medicinal herbs.

He causes the grass to grow for the cattle, and herb for the service of man: that he may bring forth food out of the earth. Psalm 104:14

Bible Clean Animals List

Buffalo Cattle Deer Reindeer Antelope Gazelles Goats
Rams Sheep
Elks Moose Caribou Giraffes

Birds

Chickens Turkeys Partridges Sparrows Doves
Pheasants Quail

Fish

Trout Tuna fish Salmon Halibut Bluegills Sunfish

Cod fish Flounder Perch Herring Sardines Bass Smelt
Mackerels

"You shall not eat any abomination.

These are the animals you may eat: the ox, the sheep, the goat, the deer, the gazelle, the roebuck, the wild goat, the ibex, the antelope, and the mountain sheep. Every animal that parts the hoof and has the hoof cloven in two and chews the cud, among the animals, you may eat. Yet of those that chew the cud or have the hoof cloven you shall not eat these: the camel, the hare, and the rock badger, because they chew the cud but do not part the hoof, are unclean for you. And the pig, because it parts the hoof but does not chew the cud, is unclean for you. Their flesh you shall not eat, and their carcasses you shall not touch.

"Of all that are in the waters you may eat these: whatever has fins and scales you may eat. And whatever does not have fins and scales you shall not eat; it is unclean for you.

"You may eat all clean birds. But these are the ones that you shall not eat: the eagle, the bearded vulture, the black vulture, the kite, the falcon of any kind; every raven of any kind; the ostrich, the nighthawk, the sea gull, the hawk of any kind; the little owl and the short-eared owl, the barn owl and the tawny owl, the carrion vulture and the cormorant, the stork, the heron of any kind; the hoopoe and the bat. And all winged insects are unclean for you; they shall not be eaten. All clean winged things you may eat.

Deuteronomy 14:3-20

The Bible meat guidelines are easy to understand. For land animals to be considered clean, they must both chew the cud and have a divided or cloven hoof. Some animals chew the cud but do not have a cloven hoof. Others have a cloven hoof but do not chew the cud. These are considered unclean. Sea life must have both scales and fins. In the Bible, fish often represent individual men and the sea represents entire populations Rev 17:15. Scales are analogous to protective armor or defensive devices. Generally, birds that forage are clean whereas birds of prey and scavengers like vultures are not. Birds are often used to represent the spiritual realm and unclean birds, sometimes, represent unclean spirits.

Chew the Cud and Cloven Hoof

An animal that "chews the cud" simply re-chews plant foods that it has already partially digested in some way. This method of nutrient absorption extracts the ultimate benefit from nutrient-poor vegetation like grass and leaves.

The principle method of chewing the cud is a process called rumination. Some animals have multiple stomachs and digest their food in stages. In the primary stages, the easily digested food and liquids are separated from the more fibrous portion and passed along the digestive tract. The courser portion, called the cud, is regurgitated and further masticated. This mixes the cud with saliva and continues to break it down into more readily absorbed nutrients.

If you have ever seen a cow or other animal casually chewing and slobbering profusely, then you have likely seen an animal chewing the cud. Animals that chew the cud in this way are called ruminants.

Not all ruminants are clean, but all clean mammals are ruminants. To be considered clean, a ruminant must also divide the hoof into two segments or toes. Each segment must terminate with a tough hoof substance. This is called a cloven hoof. Cloven hoofed mammals are quite agile on rugged or uneven terrains. This is extremely helpful to mountain goats and rams for example.

Bible Meat - Clean Animal Varieties

Most of the clean meat we consume is from the bovadae family of mammals. Cattle, goats and antelope are all bovids. They are distinguished in that the males (and sometimes females) have horns that are not branched. Some examples of bovids are cows, sheep, buffalo, mountain goats, antelope, bison and the like. Cervidae, the deer family, is distinguished by branched horns or antlers. Some examples are deer, caribou, elk, moose, mule deer, reindeer and the like. A pronghorn is also considered to be a clean animal.

In Bible symbolism and prophecy, horns represent authority and are tokens of power. Anyone who has witnessed two rams battling for supremacy can understand the metaphor.

Scavengers and Predators

It may not require much willpower to resist eating bats or vultures, but we may have trouble to resist eating pork, lobster, shellfish, catfish and other unclean meat. It is easy to reason that so many others eat these foods seemingly with no adverse effect. So what is the problem? We do not always see the rationale behind God's restrictions immediately. Similarly, we do not always justify the restrictions we place on our children. They simply trust our knowledge and experience because they understand we are interested in their welfare, and they will understand with maturity.

God does not restrict these unclean animals arbitrarily. The matter is related directly to our sanctification. As Our Creator, God is infinitely acquainted with every detriment to the most minute cell in our body. "Are not two sparrows sold for a cent? And yet not one of them will fall to the ground apart from your Father. But the very hairs of your head are all numbered. So do not fear; you are more valuable than many sparrows." Matthew 10:29-31. Our bodies are the temple of the Holy Spirit and the Spirit searches all things, yes, the deep things of God. 1 Corinthians 2:10

Many unclean animals are predators, whereas a clean animal is an herbivore. The Bible has established that every green herb was the diet originally intended for animals. When the Bible says green herb, it does not mean grain. Green herbs provide the nutrients to form muscle and flesh in these species. If we choose to eat meat, it makes sense that we eat meat formed directly from plant life and not many times removed.

Other unclean animals are scavengers. Their function is to remove putrefying carcases and filth from our lands and waters. These animals are often parasite ridden. In the case of pork and swine, the parasites can be killed by thoroughly cooking the meat, but that is not a consolation. The problem is more than parasites. The problem lies within the very constitution of the meat. If we are what we eat, then so are scavengers. Not only should we not eat them, we should not even touch the dead carcase.
They shall be an abomination to you; you shall not eat their flesh, but you shall regard their carcasses as an abomination. Leviticus 11:11

Unclean Meat

Many beef producers add growth hormones to cattle feed. Those hormones are passed along directly to the consumer's body. Some have even mingled manure and unusable carcase portions of cattle back into the feed to reduce costs and increase profits. These acts against nature make unclean animals from clean. Imagine a cow thoroughly ruminating on itself or its kind. Such detestable practices are generally considered to be the cause of Bovine Spongiform Encephalopathy, or BSE (mad cow's disease). Here are some references on the subject:
There is strong evidence and general agreement that the outbreak was amplified by feeding rendered bovine meat-and-bone meal to young calves. USDHW Addendum: This resource was removed, but the conclusion may be found here in the first paragraph: Mad Cow

Epidemiological studies conducted in the UK suggest that the source of BSE was cattle feed prepared from bovine tissues, such as brain and spinal cord, that was contaminated by the BSE agent. WHO

The point is that only eating meat deemed to be clean in Leviticus is not enough. God gave us the power of discernment. We are to make a distinction between the clean and unclean. This cannot be overstated. We see a rising trend in unsafe meat production these days. As a society, we are secreting away our elderly who are unceremoniously diagnosed with dementia or Alzheimer's disease at alarming rates. Bible health and common sense dictates, to the best of our abilities, we should know the source and quality of the meat we eat. This includes fish and poultry. If chickens are raised in over-populated coups or fish drawn from mercury- polluted waters, they should not be eaten.

I hope by reading what is written on these pages will help you with your everyday food intake. I know that by following the Bible and the ways of Jesus your life will be so much healthier.

God has a plan for each of our lives and through the Bible we can clearly see how He has laid it all out for us to follow.

With much prayer and meditating on the Word of God we will learn to do for others but also our own lives will be enriched so much more.

I wanted to put this book together to help those who had questions like I had.. I pray that you will benefit from it.

Hannah House
Publishing

Lighthouse Internatonal Ministries
MPO Box 2813
Niagara Falls, New York
14302